A Genial Senior's Companion To Ageing

PETER BUCKMAN has written books, plays, scripts for film, television and radio and has been involved in the publishing industry for many years, on both sides of the Atlantic, setting up his own literary agency when he was in his 60s.

A Genial
Senior's
Companion
To Ageing

PETER BUCKMAN

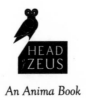

An Anima Book

This book was first published in the the UK in 2018 by Anima,
an imprint of Head of Zeus Ltd.

9 7 5 3 1 2 4 6 8

A catalogue record for this book is available from
the British Library.

ISBN (HB): 9781788540308
ISBN (E): 9781788540292

Typeset by Adrian McLaughlin

Printed and bound in Great Britain by
CPI Group (UK) Ltd, Croydon CR0 4YY

Head of Zeus Ltd
First Floor East
5–8 Hardwick Street
London EC1R 4RG

WWW.HEADOFZEUS.COM

For my grandchildren, Michael and Emma,

who have so much to look forward to.

I am in my mid-seventies, happily married to the same woman for nearly fifty years, proud parent of two daughters and grandparent of two children who are the most beautiful, intelligent and creative creatures in the known universe. I've had a reasonably successful career as a publisher and writer, and am still working as a literary agent; I'm active and healthy, despite two forms of cancer; we own the house we've lived in for forty-five years in a beautiful Oxfordshire village; and my only brush with the law, apart from going on demonstrations, was when I was busted for speeding. And yet I need reassurance. Probably we all do. Maybe it's part of our instinctive reactions: when confronted with a threat we freeze, fight, flee – or offer reassurance. And we wouldn't have lasted this long if our instincts weren't reliable.

But how do you access your instincts when they're encrusted with experience? You get yourself a book that shares the thoughts, exposes the fears, and celebrates at least some of the actions you have hitherto kept to yourself. It's no surprise that the earliest bestsellers were guides to etiquette, sex and cooking: these are areas of life where we want to give pleasure as well as receiving it, and we want to be reassured that we're doing things properly. Yet while there are endless books on how to raise our kids, there are precious few on how to embrace the ageing process. Which, considering how many there are of us seniors – so many we're a threat to the welfare budgets – is a little surprising.

We don't think we're old until suddenly we can't do something that until now has never been a problem. We don't feel we're old because our habits and reactions were formed when we were younger, and as they served us well we see no reason to change them. But we're not immune to new ideas, we're always open to persuasion, we retain our curiosity about the latest discovery and our willingness to learn. Don't we? We don't want to be lectured or patronized or told how we should behave by people who don't know what they're talking about – so why should you listen to a white middle-class male who is a Jewish atheist vegetarian socialist with republican leanings? Because you, like me, want reassurance too.

There are no prescriptions in this book, which is a personal gallimaufry of snapshot descriptions, opinions, remembrances, suggestions, and the occasional exhortation. If you believe that civility, good manners and good humour are what keep us going, I hope you will enjoy, recognize and be reassured by these entries. Incidentally, I've used the words 'I', 'you', and 'we' indiscriminately, assuming we have in common many of the experiences described. If not, I apologize, but I'm afraid there's no money-back guarantee.

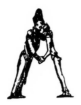

Advice should be dispensed only when requested. Of course we know a million times more than the younger generation, otherwise we've wasted an awful lot of years, but even though we're bursting with wisdom that will change everyone's lives for the better, drowning people in it will only make them splutter with indignation. Advice is like chocolate, and should be offered sparingly. My father used to say: 'Get the best advice you can, then do the opposite.' A subversive view, but worth considering.

A Genial Senior's Companion To Ageing

Age can be a bit of a problem for us seniors: if you tell people how old you are they'll think you're either lying or fishing for compliments. Or, worse, use it as a trigger to launch the 'organ recital' of all the ailments (*q.v.*) they've endured or overcome on the way to being (probably) a few years younger than you are. The thing is, nobody prepares you to behave appropriately for your age, as very few of us feel we're as old as we are. Of course our bodies remind us we can't leap about like we used to, but though we may recognize that we are old, or older, at least in the eyes of the young, few of the virtues we thought would accrue with age have materialized. Do you feel grown-up now you're past seventy? Of course not. Are you more patient, tolerant, forgiving and mellow? Yeah, right. When you're stuck behind someone strictly observing the speed limit, do you mutter approvingly? Really? Do you act more responsibly than you did when you were younger? Only if you need to reassure your children and grandchildren. One thing age does is make you a better actor.

My mother knew how to deal with age. She would never mention how old she was until she was well into her nineties (and she continued to have her hair dyed a fiery red until after her 100th birthday). One day, a much younger neighbour told her how lovely she looked. She told him he looked lovely too, to which he replied he could never hope to look as elegant as she did. 'How kind,' she said. 'I suppose I'm not bad for ninety-seven.' 'Ooh,' he countered, 'a woman who'll tell you her age will tell you anything.' My mother leaned forward conspiratorially. 'What would you like to know?' she asked.

Ailments form the content of the 'organ recital' of everything that's wrong with us, with which we regale our friends, unless they get in first. We naturally feel sympathy for someone who's got a crippling, debilitating or fatal disease, but most of us secretly draw an invisible circle around them and silently give thanks that we aren't similarly affected. We privately tell ourselves that the victim's past behaviour – their sexual shenanigans, their smoking and boozing – are probably to blame for their condition, and we make ourselves believe we were far more restrained.

Or maybe it's the fault of their genes, for which neither they nor we can be held responsible. Of course, if we suspect we've got something nasty we seek medical advice, but those aches and pains we wake up with – or, worse, get up with in the middle of the night – become as familiar as the layout of the room we fumble around on our way to the bathroom in the dark. Tell yourself that click in your knee is just cartilage, not cancer, and it won't stop you going for a walk. Ailments, the minor ones, are just reminders that we should respect the bodies that have served us well, at least so far.

Amateurs used to be the proud pioneers of science and commerce until people calling them-selves professionals claimed that a modern society needed specially trained experts to manage matters efficiently. As these same experts have made a com-plete bollocks of everything from the economy to the environment, the stock of amateurs – people like us who worked out the best way of doing things for ourselves – has risen somewhat. I'm not saying our views on the exchange rate will be taken any more seriously than our attempts at grouting tiles, but at a time when we are overwhelmed by ignorance and incompetence, we amateurs should retain the courage to speak out and contribute our two-bits' worth.

Ambition is something you should cultivate even if you've long ago retired from full-time work and boast, when drunk, depressed or seeking sympathy, that you've achieved all the goals you once set yourself. Without something to aim for you risk getting bored, and boredom (*q.v.*) is what kills you. An ambition should be just (but not too far) beyond your reach, and within your grasp if you can grab it without doing yourself an injury. Now you're a comfortable age you can rule out being the fastest, richest, best-looking or most powerful person on the planet, but you can still do your daily walk a bit quicker, or fill in the crossword or sudoku faster, or cook a dish you've never tried before to impress your friends. You can lobby to become chair of a committee you're on, because you know you'd handle it better than the incumbent. You could do things you've never got around to, like playing jazz piano or mastering mah-jong, and once you've acquired the basics you'll play to win because you've never really lost the competitive spirit that keeps you going. You may say you have, but you know yourself better than that. Ambition means looking forward, and that's got to be better than looking back.

Anger can be a wonderful release but, like all indulgences, it should be saved for special occasions. It's fine to express your irritation at politicians, foreign dictators, writers with whom you violently disagree, overacting thespians, people who stop dead in front of you to jab at their phones, and stupidity in all its forms, but if you succumb to rage with those dear to you, you may feel better, but it will only be temporary. Though we would never admit it publicly, age gnaws away at our previously held conviction that we are always in the right. I waited until I was forty to have a serious shouting match with my father, who was behaving like an arse when we were all on holiday in their house in the south of France, probably because he resented being removed from day-to-day responsibility for the firm he'd founded. Our row began when he accused me of not helping enough to entertain their guests, and it escalated to the point when I told him we would never again stay with them. At first I felt grown-up, independent, principled and courageous, but then I began to feel I'd orphaned myself, and missed the flypaper embrace of the family I grew up in, the comfort of customs that are both appealing and appalling. The cause of my anger shrank into insignificance, and it occurred to me that I might have overreacted. We made up when meeting around the hospital bed of my sister, who had just given birth to her first child, and the row was never again referred to. Anger directed at those who are closest to you may be cathartic, but the changes you hoped your shouting would bring about almost never occur. Maturity brings doubt, and once you start to think you might have acted wrongly, you will suffer insomnia and indigestion until you are reconciled.

Apologies: sorry, but you're going to have to learn to apologize, and sooner rather than later. My wife maintained that I was incapable of saying 'sorry', because I couldn't openly admit I was wrong, but age has changed that, at least a little. Occasionally, and either under unbearable provocation or the influence of drink, you may behave badly towards someone – being rude or boorish or simply ill-mannered – and if, when the mist has receded, you accept that you acted like an oaf, then, as a reasonable and grown-up person, I am sure you will see the need for an apology. You may offer it grudgingly or generously, and it may or may not be accepted, but at least you've made the gesture, and if they choose to reject it, that's their problem. But it's much harder to apologize for something you've blurted out when you're in an argument, or just a heated discussion, and your back's to the wall. At such moments your tongue leapfrogs your brain and you say something truly hurtful. I'm not talking about insisting on something as fact that later proves to be fiction: maturity means graciously accepting you may have made a mistake. Much harder to apologize for, and much harder for the abused party to accept, is the hot-tongued insult, the personal criticism that is so wounding because both of you are jolted into wondering if it reflects your true feelings. On such occasions apologies go unheeded, and it can take an astonishingly long time before the abused person is persuaded you really didn't mean it. You can always find excuses for your behaviour, such as drink (again), or a combination of frustration and instability caused by stress that resulted in temporary mental aberration which you deeply regret, but your apology, however heartfelt, will need to be backed by genuinely good behaviour for an appreciable period before it will be accepted as sincere. Sorry, but there it is.

Appearance is vitally important because it's what others judge you on. The first impression the eye sends to the brain decides in an instant what someone thinks of you, and however witty or rich or fascinating you are, you're going to have to work really hard to overcome a negative view formed by a ladder in your tights or snot on your tie. To be free of vanity you have to be a saint or an eccentric, and while it may be virtuous not to care how you look, very few of us look good without a bit of help. Beautiful people, in my experience, rarely accept or acknowledge their special quality – indeed, they often deny it. The rest of us may not aspire to beauty, or be able to rely on natural elegance to face the world with confidence, but the experience and self-knowledge that our years confer means accepting that it takes us a while to get ready properly. Those who enjoy a supportive relationship may let their partner decide which clothes go best together; otherwise you have to check your instincts by looking in the mirror. Some of us become colour-blind with age, and insist with increasing vehemence that things don't clash when your partner says they do. If you can't find an independent arbitrator – a grandchild won't do, as they shouldn't be dragged into domestic disputes – I suggest you climb down with what grace you can muster. If you're going out together, they won't want to be seen with someone who has no sense of style, will they?

A

Appetite for food, sex or new experience does not diminish with age. When good food and wine are put in front of me, I will carry on eating and drinking until either I or they are forcibly removed, whereas my wife can control her impulses, say she is full, and be strong-minded enough to refuse further helpings. Our younger daughter, who had eating disorders, has suggested I leave a little bit on my plate to tell my brain that I've had enough, but I find I'm incapable of such self-discipline. I sometimes claim it's because I was born during the Second World War, when food was rationed and if I didn't finish everything on my plate I was reminded, by hungry relatives who had probably given up some of their ration to ensure I was properly fed, that the world was full of starving children who would be glad to have my leftovers. In my formative years I went to a boys-only school where if you didn't hoover up everything quickly, someone else would nick your portion. But I accept that I am greedy and eat too much too fast because I enjoy it. Of course it leads to an expanding waistline and of course I should train myself to have smaller portions and chew everything thirty times (which supposedly fools the brain into thinking you're full, besides making the food easier to digest), and wait twenty minutes before helping myself to chocolate, but sadly the only thing that stiffens my resolve is severe stomach ache. Weighing responsibility against temptation, where food is concerned the latter is an easy winner, whereas with sex, at least for an ageing male, the parts that connect appetite to action are often so unreliable that temptation can be resisted.

Approval: as a plant needs water, we need approval from our partners, friends, colleagues, people we work with and people who work for us. Children want their parents' approval, but they don't often realize that their parents want their approval too, along with their love and respect (we don't ask too much, do we?). Religious zealots want the approval of their god, politicians want the approval of the electorate, even blood-soaked tyrants want the approval of their supporters, though the latter are terrorized into giving it. The danger for us seniors is that we know from long experience how to gain approval, and we end up doing it from habit rather than conviction. When someone we respect – a friend we haven't seen for a while, or a guru at whose feet we once sat – points out how we have changed and lost our youthful fire, compromising our principles, agreeing with theories we used to attack, or being polite to someone who deserves to be roundly criticized, we are outraged. We will say that life is too short to fight every battle, that being pragmatic is more effective than pacing the windy moral high ground, that we have learned over the years that there are some people whose views we will never change. But of course, if we simply admitted our critic was right, and that all we really wanted was for everyone to like us, they might call us pathetic, but they'd have to approve of our honesty (*q.v.*).

Arousal can still surprise us, and that's got to be a good thing. An image, a photograph, a body whose owner is proud of the work they've put into it, a dancer or an athlete showing muscular grace, the memory of an ecstatic coupling, the touch of a lover that promises nothing but is freighted with possibility: these things can arouse desire without the obligation of performance. I'm not suggesting we're no longer capable of sexual fulfilment, only that if, as I hope, we all have a full bank of memories, that gives us a generous amount of credit we needn't expend all at once. If pornography (*q.v.*) is arousal for instant gratification, there is a more thoughtful and subtle form of arousal that sets the wires of experience crackling with energy without the need to come in a neon starburst.

Attitude, like ambition *(q.v.),* is an essential attribute for an active senior, for it defines us. If you don't keep up with current developments and take a view on them, people (especially the young) will think you don't know or don't care about things that matter to them, and they will consider you out of touch, which is an insult to your knowledge and intelligence. Adopt a listening pose and it gives you licence to expound. Once you get going you can be opinionated, provided you restrain yourself from pointing out how little they know. Even if you don't win the argument or make any converts, if you can articulate your attitude you stand a reasonable chance of being taken seriously.

———

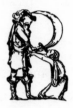

Bad behaviour is our way of showing that we can still shock, surprise, and kick against what others expect of us, but we know, and have always known, the difference between that and behaviour that is criminal. In our youth we may have tried shoplifting to gain acceptance by a gang, but that didn't lead to a career in burglary, any more than a drunken fumble led to rape: we understood the meaning of the word 'no', even if we also knew of sexist pigs who abused their power and position to commit criminal acts. You don't forget the difference between right and wrong when you grow old, and it would be a tragedy if we let others' crimes stop us being provocative, outrageous, flirtatious or rude when the occasion demands it. That way blandness lies.

Beauty can be described as an arrangement of features, whether natural or contrived – in a face, a body, a landscape, a painting, a piece of writing or music – that stirs up an instinctive sense of appreciation. The effect is not something you think about; it simply happens, though of course different things affect different people in different ways. I find beauty in a sunlit wold, you might find it in a mountainous crag that would give me vertigo, but what matters is what, if anything, we do about it. Beauty ought to be celebrated when there is so much ugliness around, but gallantry can be mistaken for predation, and wisdom dictates that you limit your compliments to those you know will appreciate them.

Bereavement is something nobody can prepare for. My mother died at 103 but it took me a long while to feel the sadness that seemed appropriate – indeed, when people called to express their condolences, I felt I was letting them down by not grieving as much as they expected. Doubtless that's because my mother went through a long decline, and her death was a relief to her and to her children, but though I miss her I only cried for her when mourning the death of a friend's daughter. When my father died, suddenly and unexpectedly, at eighty-one, I tried and failed to squeeze some tears out, but they didn't flow naturally until several months later, when I saw a Chinese film that must have reminded me of his passion for that country, and perhaps the combination of memory, love and bereavement led me to sob bitterly all the way home.

Crying, of course, is an emotional reaction over which we have little control, like that rapidly suppressed flash of glee that bubbles up when you hear of a death, not because you're glad someone's gone, but because you're relieved to be still around. You'd think that at our age we'd have had enough experience to know how to cope with death. And you'd be wrong, because you can never tell how it will take you.

Of course, the death of a child, or the person you've been loving and living with for many joyful years, is such an appalling prospect you can't armour yourself against it. The mature reaction to such a loss is not to *pretend* you know how to deal with it, but to wait until it happens and then cope with as much dignity as you can muster. Some analysts say a child is mature only when it accepts that its parents will eventually die. Now we are all living for so much longer, maybe our children will be relieved as well as saddened by our deaths, as I was at my mother's. So to hell with behaving as other people expect when mourning: let's go with our instincts, whether they involve snot or stoicism, and trust that when it's our turn we too will be properly missed, however people choose to show it.

Betrayal: we, of course, would never betray a confidence, let alone someone we loved – though sometimes I have let slip a tiny secret, unimportant and unlikely to cause harm because it would have come out anyway, and besides I was among friends and had taken a glass or two and simply forgot that I was supposed to keep it to myself. Which is totally different from, say, being tortured by nasty people to reveal details of an operation with which I might have some vague connection: not being heroic enough to withstand pain, of course I'd tell them whatever they wanted to hear. Sometimes, however, people of our generation are betrayed by someone close – a partner, a lover, even a spouse. We hope we have reached the stage when our serious relationships are not only stable but taking us together through waters that, despite an occasional storm, are relatively calm, certainly compared to our earlier years. And then something happens that is totally unexpected and devastating, the sort of thing you read about – 'wife leaves husband for childhood sweetheart after forty years of marriage' – and it's a betrayal so immense and so humiliating no one will believe you when you say you never saw it coming. Adultery is a betrayal of a relationship, and comes from the same root as corrupting or diluting something. When a friend of ours suffered from this catastrophe, we all rallied round, and were soon introducing him to new people as though he were divorced or widowed. The trouble was, he couldn't believe he had been guilty of doing anything that provoked the betrayal, whether it was some casual infidelity that had come to light, or some act of selfishness that had led to festering resentment. Eventually he found someone else, but we were concerned that if he'd learned nothing from the experience, it might be repeated. Betrayal blows up your very foundations, and as you can't build on rubble, you have to dig deep to create something new.

Birthdays are occasions I take very seriously. I know many prefer to avoid commemorating the passing of the years, as merely reciting the numerals makes them feel ancient. For me, they are an opportunity to celebrate being alive despite occasional illness, frequent disappointment, periodic frustration, and my inability to persuade people that a civilized polity is possible if only they were sensible and shared my beliefs. In a good year, birthdays offer proof that despite being an age I would once have regarded as totally decrepit, I don't entirely look it, and can certainly behave childishly. I love surprises (they keep you on your toes) and my family know that and generously surprise me. And, of course, birthdays are an opportunity to be generous in a personal and thoughtful way. It's not the gifts – the older we get, the less clutter most of us want – it's the act of making contact, choosing a card, organizing a gathering, toasting survival. Birthdays are individual occasions, free from the commercialization of high holidays like Christmas or manufactured obligations like Mothers' Day. I like to celebrate mine at least three times – once in anticipation, once on the actual day, once to postpone the feeling it's all over and may never be repeated. Far from keeping our birthdays quiet, I think we should enjoy them as vigorous proof of our continuing presence, being generous to our friends and enjoying the annoyance of our enemies.

Book groups are a form of social intercourse that can be intellectually stimulating, while being (usually) less competitive than bridge parties. You get to see other people's houses, maybe drink their wine and nibble their canapés, meet new people, diplomatically rubbish their taste (at least in books), and read something you would never normally pick up. Most members are women, and their literary interests are usually more adventurous than men's – one group I know read all three volumes of *Fifty Shades of Grey* while their male partners concentrated on a history of the Peninsular War. On the other hand, when it's your turn to act as host you have to clean to exceptional standards, prepare (or buy) morsels that are dainty and distinctive without making you look like a show-off, and offer wine better than you would normally imbibe. And then you have to think of a book for everyone to read next time, which involves a great deal of research, in addition to having intelligent comments to make about the work you're there to discuss, which you've hardly had time to look at, given all the other burdens of hospitality. Also, over time the other members' views can become predictable, they interrupt just when you're developing a point or, worse, they say what you were going to say before you can articulate it. And though everyone is a volunteer, forcing yourself to read a new book every month somehow smacks of being made to do your homework, with virtue often being eclipsed by resentment. But then, what other than a book can get you out of the house, charge up your brain, and lead you to encounter new faces, new ideas and new writers?

Boredom can be fatal. Being a wage slave may have been boring, but that was the tedium of the routine. Hopefully the work had some point, and at least you were regularly rewarded. Boredom is when you don't have the mental energy to set yourself goals or follow a routine that gets you nearer to achieving them. It's like being ill: you can't operate at full throttle, you mope around until you feel better, but you'll never feel better if at the end of the day you've nothing to show for your suffering. It isn't having nothing to do – that problem can be solved with drink or other distractions. It's having nothing to do that seems enjoyable or worthwhile. Mowing the lawn is boring, but the result is pleasing, so the effort pays off. You can spend days trying to build or decorate or even compose something that doesn't come right, but you persevere because you get a kick out of it, or at least learn from the experience. Boredom is when nothing seems inviting, enticing or engaging; when you've lost control of your imagination and ambition and feel like giving up. Like depression *(q.v.)* and other debilitating states of mind, you have to realize what's happening and make the decision to change it. Nobody else can do it for you.

———

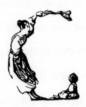

Calories should, we are frequently told, be counted religiously if we want to keep fit and avoid obesity. Which is fine if you like making lists *(q.v.)* and you're obsessive about weighing your portion of breakfast muesli and consulting your guide so that you can give yourself the joyous news that you've got 1,894 calories left for the rest of your day – but can you rely on the guide's accuracy? We've lived through enough changes of 'expert opinion' to be mistrustful: if eggs are bad for you one week and good for you the next, can we be confident that the number of calories they supposedly contain is scientifically precise? Of course we all cheat a little on our own, 'forgetting'

to count that tiny bit of butter that would otherwise go to waste, splashing a bit more gin into our glass that takes it over the 'standard' measure, but how were those figures printed in bright colours on labels arrived at? When car manufacturers cheat on their emission and consumption figures, are food and drink manufacturers immune? Just worrying about this question probably uses as many calories as a brisk walk, because the brain expends an amazing amount of energy, but who adds that to the reckoning? Let's face it, if you're going to obsess about your calories, it's best to embrace your competitive side and join a fitness programme, because doing it on your own is (a) ineffectual, as you're bound to lose patience and cheat, and (b) rather sad.

Caution creeps up on you. We've all learned, over the years, to be cautious about things like weather or economic forecasts, the opinions of so-called experts, members of the opposite sex who insist they want a no-strings relationship, and anyone who offers the investment of a lifetime. But there's a difference between being cautious about advice and cautious about action. Say someone proposes you accompany them on an adventure holiday in a place you've never visited. When you were young you would have accepted without a second thought, right? Now, you weigh up the disadvantages – the cost, the tedium of getting there, the dangers and discomfort of roughing it in a place unprepared for tourism, the amount of pills and potions you'll have to pack and the risk of running out of essential supplies – and you think, fuck it, I'd rather stay at home. On the one hand you are conserving your resources and will probably live longer by avoiding bandits and mysterious infections, on the other you are depriving yourself of an experience that could enhance your life with a jolt of the unusual. Being sensible about taking risks is one thing, being cautious about the unexpected may verge on cowardice *(q.v.)*. It's the perennial conflict between instinct and intellect that we all have to face, with one consolation: if we err on the side of caution, at our age we are used to living with regret *(q.v.)*.

Celebrations of an old friend's life, whether they're living or dead, are like that extra bit of chocolate: you grab at it greedily, knowing you'll probably regret it afterwards. You accept an invitation to a memorial because you want to pay tribute and comfort the family, and also because you want privately to celebrate your own survival and see how you compare to those contemporaries who are left. But when you've schlepped yourself over to wherever the event is taking place, complaining at the cost and difficulty of getting there when you'd be much more comfortable at home, where your own wine is far superior to that served at the party, and knowing there'll never be enough food worth eating, you encounter all the problems involved in facing up to your past. People look vaguely familiar but you can't remember their names and think it's rude to ask. When you introduce yourself they can't hear you, so you have to shout; they look blank, but announce their own name, which you can't quite catch. If you do find someone you know, you quickly discover there's very little to talk about once you've lied about them not having changed, and exchanged lists of ailments (*q.v.*). If it's a large party the noise is deafening, the speeches inaudible, and you wonder who all these young people are who couldn't possibly have known your aged friend, and while some of them may talk politely to you, they have no idea of your reputation and probably are only there for the booze. Old acquaintances seem to have become bent and boring, never mind losing their sense of humour: either they don't appreciate your attempt to add levity to the proceedings by making witty comments, or they're too deaf or drunk to care. The opportunity such events offer of catching up with people you once held dear can be hollow and disappointing – but of course you will go on attending them while you can, if only to show you're still around.

Celebrity is a sunbeam of recognition from gods we don't believe in. When I was young, I told myself that the thrill I got from talking to somebody famous was because they had achieved something that was beyond the reach of ordinary people, even those (like me and you) with unlimited ambition. There was a reason they had achieved celebrity status: they were the best at what they did, supreme at the summit of the mountains the rest of us were waiting to climb. Now we are more experienced, and perhaps a touch embittered after getting a little lost on our way to the top, we can be grateful at not being celebrities, and be at ease in their company. When once we mocked their desire for privacy, and told ourselves we could cope with the scalding heat of fame as long it was accompanied by a reasonable fortune and the ability to get a table in fashionable restaurants, now we mock their frequently chronicled failings, pity their inability to sustain lasting relationships, agree with those who ascribe their success to chance or corruption or clever marketing rather than talent, and unworthily rejoice when their reputations are shredded. We'd still have dinner with them, though. A fallen angel still has wings.

Chance and luck *(q.v.)* are different, in my opinion. Chance begins a process, luck plays a part in completing or defeating it. You can't rely on chance, but you can make your own luck: chance may afflict you with an awful disease, luck – and getting the right medical attention – may see you cured. Experienced people like us should be able to recognize luck, in the sense of it being an opportunity, but only a wild optimist, bordering on fantasist, would count on being rescued by chance, in the sense of the random operation of forces beyond our understanding. The trouble is few of us learn from our own mistakes, let alone other people's, and we persist in confusing the various meanings of chance in the hope of getting out of trouble. We welcome a chance meeting that leads to new opportunities as a sign of fate being on our side; if it all goes pear-shaped, even the most mature of us is apt to deny responsibility and blame factors outside our control. We all know, and tell others, that things shouldn't be left to chance, but that doesn't stop us doing just that. It's a sign of our gambling nature, and possibly our laziness, but assuming we've avoided plunging our families into destitution, we will doubtless continue to avoid practising what we preach.

C

Change is difficult and uncomfortable, but that doesn't mean we should avoid it. It can be forced on us by unexpected circumstances: an accident, an illness, or a malfunction in a machine we rely on, such as a car or computer. If your partner suddenly breaks a leg and needs you to abandon your usual activities to take care of them, you're going to show what an adaptable, tolerant, responsible person you are, and change accordingly. The odd thing is, the older we get the more we grumble about change, yet we often face the greatest change of all, from independence to dependence, with little or no preparation. I suppose it's because it's something we don't want to think about too much, as we're secretly confident we'll cope when we have to. Like always.

Charity can be immensely satisfying if you're working for one or supporting a worthy (and effective) charitable organization with your philanthropic donations, but it can consume you with guilt when you've not got much money and are deluged with requests for help. One elderly woman killed herself because she couldn't cope with the sheer volume of competing demands from good causes, but that shouldn't stop us giving altogether. Charity contributes to our well-being: it allows most of us to feel better about ourselves for a relatively small outlay and very little effort. When you see pictures of individual victims of war, famine, natural disaster, birth defects, epidemics or simple poverty, your instinct is to offer them money. You know that some of it will be siphoned off by corrupt officials, that the aid it buys will be exploited by criminals, and anyway won't be nearly enough to help all those in need, but even so it's better than doing nothing. Charity is a poor way of righting the wrongs of the world, but the victims deserve our support, as do the people who work for them, if only because there is little chance we'd go out and do what they're doing.

Children: you knew you were doing something right when your children moaned at you for being so restrictive, and your parents gently (but pointedly) criticized you for letting your offspring run wild.

C

Now we are grandparents we can spoil our grandchildren with impunity, but how do we develop a
relationship with our offspring that is supportive,
tolerant, and resilient enough to withstand the inevi-
table rows? Especially when they move back in with
us because they can't afford a place of their own,
or they've lost their job or broken up a relationship
and have nowhere else to go. We're glad to see them,
of course, and for a while their presence makes a
welcome change. But when the new routines (*q.v.*)
we have established as 'empty nesters' are interrupted
or disregarded, and the spaces we have taken over
are suddenly occupied, while we love our children
and are full of sympathy for their predicament,
it's hard to avoid just a touch of resentment and
frustration at the way we're being used. Doubtless
they feel the same.

Our generation prides itself on having a very
different, and much warmer, relationship with our
own children than our parents had with us. We set
boundaries for our kids to bounce off, we tried not
to make threats that we couldn't or wouldn't carry
out, but perhaps the biggest difference was that we

explained the reasons for the rules we wanted them to observe, rather than simply laying them down. My childhood relationship with my parents was based on me accepting their authority, my relationship with our children was based on justifying whatever authority I wielded. If we can move on from the fact that our parents' behaviour towards us was irritating, unfair, and often irrational, and accept that they were far from perfect but convinced they were doing their best, we should try and persuade our own children to see us too as loving but flawed. When they're young, children want their parents to be infallible; by the time they're teenagers they know we often make mistakes; when they're adults we must hope the mistakes they may have made help them to regard us more tolerantly, especially if they're sharing our space. Closeness means you can confront your problems together, which is some compensation for the strain caused by enforced proximity.

Chores are jobs you want to get out of the way so you can do something more creative, but they can

C

also give you a sense of achievement. None of us wants them to define our day: we have moved on from the time when routine tasks, such as the housework that was expected of women when we were young, are considered fulfilling in themselves. Now that we have reached the age when we don't have to clock in to work or answer to bosses or do jobs we know are beneath or beyond us, we are entitled to take a break and do little or nothing once we've laid the table, sorted out the fire or boiler, and dealt with the washing. The trouble is that doing little or nothing soon strengthens the acid of puritan guilt (*q.v.*). We bring in the firewood or get the ironing out of the way, and then what? Why are we in such a hurry to be done with the chores when we haven't decided, or simply don't know, what to do with the rest of our time? Shouldn't we take things more slowly, to allow further plans to develop and mature? There are those who say the urge to deal with little matters quickly is a product of the internet culture, and particularly the pressure to respond instantly to emails. But it surely goes back to the time when the provider was forced to stand aside for somebody younger, and invented a list of tasks to keep themselves occupied and make them seem indispensable. We're always in a rush because we don't know what's around the corner, but if there really isn't something you're desperate to do once you've taken out the rubbish, remember that the more chores you do, the more chores there will be for you to do, and take your time.

Competing might be an evolutionary thing to ensure we survive as a species, but you would have thought that when we've reached the age of watching our grandchildren grow up, we'd stop worrying about whether our car will look as good as those of the other people collecting them from school, or whether our clothes are the right mix of hip and casual without looking flash or dowdy. We carry on competing in ways that can be subtle – 'Oh, you still go to the sales? I buy everything online' – and crude: 'I wouldn't be seen dead in one of those cut-price supermarkets, their wines are so hit-and-miss.' It seems we can't stop ourselves competing against each other, even though our place in the pecking order has long been established. Either it's a habit we can't kick, or a way of proving we still have a kick in us, that no one can take us for granted. Competing is perfectly healthy provided you don't let it become a consuming and destructive lust for a victory that is beyond your financial or physical grasp; and providing that you limit the competition to people of your own age and situation. The young will find you competing against them laughable, and everyone will find you competing against easy targets contemptible.

Confidence seems to become more brittle as you grow older. It would be nice to think that we keep it polished like a favourite pair of shoes, so that it's flexible and resistant to stains, but often an unexpected knock puts a big hole in it. Experience should make us resilient, but it doesn't matter whether you're a politician or a poet, criticism hurts and confidence suffers. We tell ourselves we should be grown-up about it and not let ourselves be affected, but what sensitive person like you or me doesn't think there might be some truth in what our critics are saying? It's taken me years to be confident that the way I think and feel is shared by enough people to justify me writing a book like this, but I hope I'm confident enough to listen to differing views, for ignoring them would be a sign of insensitivity and inflexibility. Mind you, only a saint or a tyrant maintains their confidence in the face of fierce opposition: myself, I need a good sulk and a stiff drink before my confidence levels trickle back to normal.

Conscience may soften with age, like almost everything else, but there's a thin steel core that is both flexible and indestructible. Years of using and abusing the moral code we call conscience teaches us what we can get away with, but as with bad behaviour *(q.v.)*, however much we have compromised there are still some basic things we don't do (unless we're totally depraved). Conscience is what keeps us civilized, makes us predictable to our children, acceptable to our partners, and reliable to our friends. Far from making you a moralizing bore, it's actually something to boast of and celebrate, like having your own hair and teeth.

Cooking contributes hugely to my well-being. I'm not particularly good at it, and I promise I'm not going to give you my favourite recipes, but I started to explore cooking when I became a vegetarian in my early forties, and in my mid-seventies I've found it embodies almost all the qualities that make our lives enjoyable. You can be spontaneous, inventive, even thrifty when using up food that would otherwise get thrown out. You can follow a recipe, improve on it (or ruin it), or improvise: it's the perfect occupation for the amateur and gifted dilettante (*q.v.*). Your work has a purpose and isn't just a chore *(q.v.)*, its aim is to satisfy your own appetites and, if cooking for others, to give pleasure (*q.v.*) and show off your expertise. You can go looking for particular ingredients or you can produce stuff you've actually grown. You can use the latest fancy equipment or make a virtue of simple tools, you can create a huge pile of washing-up or gain enormous credit by clearing up as you go.

You can take as much time as you need and no one will accuse you of wasting it. Cooking engages the brain, and requires a wide variety of discrete physical and intellectual skills, such as measuring, timing, chopping and slicing, mixing ingredients for anything from pastry to a roux, seasoning and tasting. It also involves a reasonable amount of exercise, and can legitimately be accompanied, and often improved, by alcohol. You can be as creative as you're capable of being, and if it all goes wrong you will get sympathy rather than censure. What's not to like?

Cowardice is something you redefine as you grow older. It's different from caution *(q.v.):* when we were young, to be cautious was a sign of sagacity, whereas to be called a coward was the greatest insult. But after decades of learning what we can and can't cope with, it doesn't seem cowardly to avoid involvement in contests we can't win, it's only putting our experience to sensible use. If, like me, you were bullied at school, you felt like a coward for not standing up for yourself, even if no one named you as such.

Having weathered the experience, and hopefully learned how to deal with similar situations in adult life, I no longer think of myself as a cowardly boy, just a survivor. Conscientious objectors in the First World War were called cowards, but eventually came to be seen as men of courage and principle. While we would all hope to protect ourselves or our families if we came under attack, avoiding heroics and pointless posturing is a sign of maturity. If gangs of macho youths are squaring up for a fight, you don't step between them, you call the police. If some drunk taunts you, you don't retaliate, you ignore them. We have all suffered humiliations, and with luck they have taught us when to retreat and when to fight back, when to negotiate and when to compromise. I think that for grown-ups, cowardice isn't running away from what others threaten to do to you, it's refusing to accept responsibility (*q.v.*) for your own actions. A small example: I was at a party given by an architect friend with a fiery wife. I saw him in close, and doubtless innocent, conversation with another woman in an adjoining room. For some drunken reason, in that mischievous, mildly malicious spirit that enjoys provoking confrontation between contented couples, I told his wife what he was up to. She marched in, smashed his guitar over his head, and marched out again. He was understandably puzzled and asked me what had provoked such an attack. Instead of telling him that I had caused it, I said I had no idea. I felt like a coward, and I still do.

Curiosity can be life-enhancing when handled with the delicacy we have acquired over the years. Showing a non-prurient interest in a complete stranger – a shop assistant or a new barperson in your local pub – and encouraging them to talk about themselves, which everyone enjoys doing, melts their professionalism into something quite friendly, once they're confident you're not a police officer or bailiff, but merely (in my case) a Harmless Old Buffer. People can surprise you and confound your expectations. I asked a guy in a phone shop about the elegant Chinese calligraphy tattooed on his arm, and he revealed it was his birth sign, a present from someone he was no longer speaking to, and to avoid negative thoughts he was going to have it covered by another tattoo, rather than having it removed. An entire life story in a brief exchange that made me feel better about humanity in general and the young in particular.

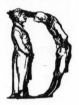

Dancing is an activity our generation is supposed to be good at. Sadly I'm not, even though I wrote a social history of dance, which was mainly plagiarized from other sources and was popular because of the illustrations. At a ninetieth birthday party I attended recently, line dancing provided the entertainment, and oldies not only outnumbered the youngsters, but outperformed them in

Even though I'm bo

everyone else is de

was evident. Of c

cise as well as h

get away with

your private parts, but comfort yourself with the thought that it's no more intimate than having your hairdresser attack the top of your head, and it's done in private rather than public.

Politeness is surely ingrained in us and oozes out regardless of any provocation to be rude. It involves taking people seriously, listening to them, and responding courteously. Nothing infuriates a young hooligan more than being treated politely, though that may lead to violence rather than an improvement in manners. When I receive cold calls just when I'm eating or watching TV, I always preface my coldly furious response with 'Sorry, but…'. In argument, the thrust of the knife is made all the more effective when delivered politely, and if it makes us look quaintly old-fashioned, or even faintly ridiculous, at least we won't be ignored.

Political correctness is a distorted image of politeness *(q.v.)*, and however absurd some of the linguistic contortions are that people go through to avoid giving offence, we have to pay it lip service. Of course, it's hard to keep up with changes in vocabulary when words we used without thinking are suddenly taboo. Authors who were popular in our parents' day use terms like 'Hebrews' or 'bolshies' or 'niggers', and apologists excuse them on the grounds that they were just reflecting the culture of their time. But those authors were actually anti-Semites, conservatives and white supremacists, whereas when tolerant and fair-minded people like us employ words that are politically incorrect we never intended to offend anyone. Nevertheless, it's worth trying to come to terms with new terminology, as new words encapsulate new attitudes, and that can sometimes be a sign of progress.

Politics see *Understanding*.

Pornography is so widely available on the internet that I'm sure every man with access to a computer has looked at it more than once. And many women too, though they usually have better things to do with their time. Being aroused by watching other people who appear to enjoy what they're doing doesn't seem perverted to me, unless what you're watching is against the law or involves coercion. If you're in a relationship, it may be considered an act of notional infidelity, though it could also be described as a flirtation with fluids that are better out than in. We all know pornography is an industry that has criminal elements and that commodifies and commercializes sex and especially women. It also gives young people an unreal image of what sex is actually like for ordinary people, those who don't have unfeasibly large breasts or huge penises. But the internet offers good stuff as well as bad, and if old people want to pleasure themselves in private watching others do the same, it surely doesn't deserve condemnation out of hand. *See also Masturbation.*

Posture matters only when you catch sight of yourself in a mirror or shop window and wonder who that poor bent old creature is. We've got so used to the way we walk, stand and sit that we imagine our heads are up, our backs straight and our shoulders square, whereas to the rest of the world we resemble an ambling turtle. We know perfectly well that slumping and slouching aren't attractive, make us look small, and enhance the unsightly bulges between our shoulders and our knees. We also know that it's really not hard to make the effort to stand tall and sit straight; what's hard is keeping it up for more than a minute or two. There's no evidence that slouching is bad for your health – I had an uncle by marriage who was a professor of anatomy and insisted that trying to keep the spine rigidly straight was unnatural as well as injurious – and your friends and loved ones are accustomed to the way you look and would be suspicious or alarmed if you suddenly started sitting straight-backed on the edge of the sofa like a Victorian dowager. Some elderly men throw back their shoulders in the presence of an attractive young person, but we all know wit and wisdom are far more enticing than a parade-ground posture that can't possibly be sustained.

P

Power, for everyone except monarchs and dictators, is something we *used* to have. In the physical sense, we can't lift or carry what we once did; and the power to command others to do our bidding has long since passed into younger hands. We may carry out traditional roles in our families, or enjoy ceremonial titles in the business we created or expanded, but being addressed as chairman when strategy is decided by the chief executive is like putting a crown on a snowman: it looks impressive, but no one takes it seriously. We are playing a part with which we, and our audience, are wearily familiar, and there's no scope to enlarge it. When the horizon is no longer within reach, you can accept it gracefully (which, unless you are saintly, will scarcely camouflage your resentment); you can bellow defiance (which will result in a lot of eye-rolling exasperation); or you can focus on smaller kingdoms over which you will rule undisputed. Put the skills and experience you have acquired over the years to unexpected use. Small is even more beautiful when you can't see as far as you once could.

Prejudices are what other people have, because they're not as open-minded, rational, tolerant, generous, educated, civilized, wise, balanced and experienced as we are. It's hard to persuade a prejudiced person to change their mind in private; in public it's impossible, and sometimes dangerous. We have learned over the years to pick the battles we think we can win, but sometimes we have to stand up and fight prejudice even though we will probably be defeated. The scars are honourable, and with any luck we will have inflicted enough damage to make them think again. Or at least reassure ourselves that our instinct for decency is not entirely dormant.

Pretending starts in childhood, and we get better at it as we grow older. But whereas children can change roles swiftly, and are quick to correct anyone who isn't playing their part properly, some of us find it increasingly hard to abandon a character we have pretended to be for so long. It's fine when you act brave to reassure someone who is frightened, or pretend to know more about a subject than you do in order to impress or win an argument – we all do that. It's when you project fantasy as reality – if, say, you pretend to be rich, or organized, when the truth is you are only just managing and your affairs are in chaos – that the danger lies. The chances are you won't be found out, if you've carried off the pretence for so many years, but if your mask slips – if, for example, you were taken ill and someone investigated your true situation – you risk your entire reputation being exploded. It doesn't take much for people envious of the character you've created to label you a fantasist, and that could undermine the genuine achievements you may have made. Pretence is addictive, and it requires real resolution to be honest about it before it's too late.

Pride is a virtue, not a vice, and we have surely earned the right to enjoy it. We are proud of what our children and grandchildren achieve, as well as the successes of our friends, provided they are balanced by the occasional failure. Why shouldn't we be proud of our own achievements, or at any rate the ones that were honourably earned, or where the dishonour has been forgotten or forgiven?

Principles: do these change as we acquire experience and wisdom? Of course they bloody do! There is a subtle difference between principles and convictions: the latter are what we believe about a particular topic, the former a set of beliefs that cover our entire behaviour. Convictions can, or should, be changed by facts – if not, they become prejudices (*q.v.*). Principles are formed by, or in reaction to, education and example, and they alter as we learn more, largely from those we love or live with. If principled behaviour is not changed by new experiences, we would never evolve and instead become the grumpy old persons of caricature. As for being models of consistency, where's the fun in that? Keeping ourselves as well as others on their toes is what ageing is all about.

Psychotherapy is big business and, like other big businesses, not always well regulated. There are professional associations for almost every activity, but having a diploma from them is not necessarily a guarantee of respectability. Yet just having somebody listen to you sympathetically is valuable, and if they encourage you to wrap words round your problems, you're on the road to coping with them. You don't have to agree with their analysis of what caused you to despair, any more than you have to go back to a physio whose manipulations made you feel worse. And though everyone you know will recommend their favourite, you know you'll go with the friend whose judgement you trust and respect.

Punctuality is a habit that's hard to break. Whether you're the infuriating type who always leaves time for emergencies, or the sort who still arrives puffing and red-faced and blaming everything but yourself for being late, that's how you've always been, and you're unlikely to change now. I hate keeping people waiting, but hate even more being kept waiting and wasting what remains of my time: as a result, I constantly hover between anger and anxiety. If I'm the guest, I think it's only polite to arrive slightly late, as if I'm the host my ambition is to be there slightly ahead of time and appear totally serene and unruffled. You'd think that at our age we'd have stopped worrying about such trifles, but it's been dinned into us that punctuality is the politeness of kings, and we either conform or rebel.

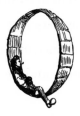

Quarrels are exhausting and unprofitable between long-term partners, especially when they go over ground that has been dug up as often as a vegetable patch. Between new partners, on the other hand, quarrels can be revealing and informative, as each stakes out ground unfamiliar to the other, and gives them a flash of the weaponry deployed against them. It's a mistake to think you can pick your quarrels: rather, they pick you, and you have to decide whether you're going to sort them out through rational discussion, ignore them and sulk, or blow on them until they flare into open warfare. If you join battle, it becomes a matter of victory or defeat, though a master of strategy should be able to persuade their opponent to surrender by making them believe they have won.

Questions should be answered seriously when they come from our grandchildren, though of course we are entitled, indeed expected, to embroider the truth. We can also be open when questioned by people who appear genuinely interested in our opinions and history, for which of us does not enjoy the opportunity to talk about themselves? Where we should be guarded, however, is when asked questions that we know will be stored and sold as marketing data. We live in a society that wants to know so much about us, their questions amount to an invasion of privacy. I don't mind ticking or filling in boxes with my name, address and date of birth in order to open an account or make a purchase, but as that should give them enough to establish my bona fides, I don't see why I should tell them where I was born, my marital state, or how I came across their services. The trouble is, they probably know these things anyway,

Q

as few of us think the answers we too readily supply will be used against us. We also tend to believe that with so much information available, the chances of us being singled out for some malign purpose are as slim as winning the lottery. We could be wrong.

———•———

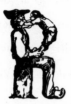

Realism is important at our age, but we shouldn't let it cramp our imagination entirely. We haven't got this far without being realistic about what does and doesn't work, and we know our limitations as well as those of the people we interact with. But being hardened by experience needn't stop us taking on a challenge: optimists will believe they'll emerge triumphant, pessimists will expect disaster, but even the most realistic of us still has dreams.

Regrets are like the stuffed toys we comforted ourselves with as children, things we should have grown out of but can't bear to throw away. We've all got much to regret, so many encounters that ended badly, the memories of which make us sit up in the middle of the night with a nightmare shudder, either because we're still owed an apology, or we didn't apologize when we could and should have. We know we shouldn't dwell on these matters, but like all the stuff we've stored out of sight, they're never quite out of mind. Of course we should have a good clear-out and face the future cleansed, but who wants to be clean and pure when the rest of the world fights dirty? However ashamed we are of the things we regret, like that scruffy old toy it's a comfort to know we can give them a private airing when we need to.

Relaxing is hard when you're as busy as we are, latecomers to a culture that insists on instant response as well as instant gratification. To relax properly is not the same as wasting time *(q.v.):* you have to be disciplined, which appears to be a contradiction in terms. You need to set aside a period of at least twenty minutes, during which you use whatever method you prefer to empty your mind and allow your body to find its natural alignment. I know that sounds like psychobabble, and I'm not good on meditation, nor have I tried yoga *(qq.v.)*, but I did find the Alexander Technique effective in easing aches and pains, and it had the additional benefit of making me less dependent on an inhaler for allergies by teaching me how to relax my chest and lungs. It didn't make me taller or more attractive, but then relaxing is about looking inward and disengaging from the usual concerns that absorb our energies and nag at our confidence.

Religion is a subject on which people of our age have long ago made up our minds, and as a Jewish atheist all I'm going to say is that the rituals for solemn events like weddings and funerals still bring people together for a common purpose, whatever their faith, and that places of worship are impressive monuments to community belief. At its best, religion offers charity to the poor, care for the sick and comfort to the lonely; at less than its best it cloaks in respectability the small-minded, the censorious, the intolerant and the fanatic.

But while a secular or humanist ceremony can equal the religious ones in emotional grandeur, they don't have the hymns, do they?

Resolutions have been broken so often during the many years we've been striving for improvement that it's a wonder we go on making them. It's a combination of habit, optimism and self-delusion: we find that a favourite garment has suddenly grown too small, and in a fit of self-disgust we resolve to give up our favourite vices, and while we're about it we'll also stop swearing or growling at our loved ones. We end up fulfilling none of those resolutions, and console ourselves by over-indulging even more, telling ourselves it doesn't really matter at our time of life, and conveniently ignoring the fact that while we're very good at criticizing a lack of willpower in others, we've learned very little about controlling our own.

Respect should be accorded us for our sheer survival, if not for our achievements. Sadly, we do not always receive our due, because there are now so many of us oldies our age is unremarkable and hardly merits attention. What can we do to gain respect, assuming that's what we want? Heroic deeds are probably beyond us, philanthropy is so common it would have to be on a massive scale, and while a sudden change of behaviour would rightly be regarded with suspicion, consistency is too boring to alter attitudes, unless you're royalty. You don't get respect by drawing attention to yourself, or if you do it doesn't last long, and though the ability to make people laugh is much respected, it's no good if you can't deliver a punchline effectively. In my view, respect is like approval and the universal desire to be loved: if you do what you enjoy as well as you can and pretend not to care what other people think, respect may be yours. Or not, but at least you're having fun.

Responsibility can't, alas, be shirked, at least not until we can no longer take responsibility for ourselves. We may frequently want to take a step back, to let others stand in the firing line, to watch from a distance while those we love ignore our advice and do things that end in tears, whether it's dissipating their emotional energy on doomed relationships or wasting their political energy on futile gestures. Of course they should act responsibly, but if they don't we can't give up on them, any more than we can turn up the thermostat and stop worrying about global warming, or pick up a plastic bottle of water and ignore the fact that it will find its way into the deepest and darkest parts of our oceans. We grew up believing the individual can and should make a difference, and just because we've done our bit doesn't, sadly, mean there isn't more to be done. However tempting it is to let others carry the torch for progress, the need for effective action is greater than ever, and because we wouldn't be where we are today if we hadn't acted responsibly at least some of the time, we owe it to ourselves to carry on.

Retirement is a nonsensical term: to call yourself 'retired' is a totally inaccurate description of all the activities and anxieties that fill your waking, and often your sleeping, hours. Just because you are no longer in full-time employment doesn't mean you have withdrawn from the world, or that you have nothing more to contribute to it. I am self-employed and still working in my seventies; the father of a friend of mine still put in a few hours most days at his desk in the City, and he was 102. Being forced to give up a job you enjoyed just because you have reached an arbitrary age is ridiculous and insulting, and a bus pass and a pension are small compensation. If we're still active, capable, and taking pride and pleasure in our work, we should be encouraged to continue.

Retirement villages, unlike retirement homes, sound quite attractive if you can afford them. You have your own living space, there are plenty of leisure activities, communal restaurants for those who can't be bothered to cook, and assistance and medical care are always available. The grounds and buildings are secure, and though your neighbours are strangers they will be of your generation and suffer from similar ailments *(q.v.)*. Unlike a retirement home, where the staff struggle to care for a disparate collection of often demented people who can't look after themselves, a retirement village doesn't operate a regime with a strict set of rules that benefit the owner rather than the occupant. But would you want to live in a community consisting only of people like you – people of similar age, income and interests? The village we live in had a properly mixed population when we bought our house, but thanks to the ridiculous rise in property prices only the seriously wealthy can now afford to buy here. Isn't the joy of living in a mixed community having children around, and young people in touch with the latest trends, even the occasional vandal to grumble about, as well as persons with different backgrounds, experiences and views that may not be the same as yours? When I get to the stage of being unable to take care of myself, I hope I'll be able to afford a carer and have family around to keep an eye on me and them. If not, I'd opt for assisted dying with dignity, but whatever the case I wouldn't want to live with people just like me: that would be boring, and boredom *(q.v.)* is what kills you.

Routines are the banisters that get us through the day. They are deeply personal, and often seem ridiculous to outsiders who have their own rituals to keep them going. You probably don't remember how or why you started on your particular routine, and assuming you don't suffer from OCD, you'd regard it as quite flexible and subject to change at whim. Routines offer a comfortable straitjacket in which you can do stuff without having to think about it, but when they start to run your life, rather than you being in charge, they've become obsessions *(q.v.)*, and need to be challenged.

Rudeness is rare at our age, unless you've got dementia or Tourette's. We allow tactlessness to pass with politeness *(qq.v.)* for the sake of a quiet life, and we would only be rude, at least outside the family, in response to an intolerable insult or act of gratuitous provocation. To be effective as well as pardonable, rudeness has to be instinctive, and is stronger if laced with wit, but if you can't manage that, you can show you're in control by staying calm. If an outburst is unstoppable, let rip and leave, preferably before they can respond.

———

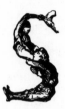

Saving is what survivors like us do instinctively. Money aside, we save things we know will come in useful, as well as things that are worth saving *just in case* they come in useful. We can't help ourselves, even though we've vowed to downsize (ridiculous word, like something Alice might do in Wonderland), and get rid of all our clutter to make it easier for our children when we've gone. It may be that we are influenced by the example of our grandparents (my grandma scrubbed tinfoil and saved it for reuse) and our parents, who stockpiled everything from loo paper to tinned food long after the war and rationing had ended. And there were no sell-by dates in those days: you kept stuff until it stank, rotted or, in the case of tins, blew its top. Though our own lives have seen the longest period of peace in Europe ever recorded, we still have the memories of war imprinted on our minds, and part of us wants to hoard stuff in case of disaster. But as our children, benign products of the age of obsolescence, won't touch stuff that's out of date, our saving is something of a wasted exercise, and they covertly or openly mock us for it. Unlike their attitude to our saving money...

Secrets are not all that safe when we grow forgetful about who we're not supposed to share them with. I'm not known for my discretion, but I can still persuade friends to tell me their secrets, because at our age gossip is as highly prized as when we were at school. There are few things more thrilling than betraying a confidence and knowing it will in turn be betrayed: it's not necessarily malicious, more like a game of pass the parcel where you want to get rid of the goods to avoid paying a forfeit. Of course, if someone younger confides in you and swears you to secrecy, you have to honour your vow, though if you suspect they might harm themselves, or others, you should be devious enough to warn those who can prevent that happening, and then protest your innocence to the one you have betrayed. They won't believe you, but it's better than saying you did it for their own good, and they might even be grateful, or you can so comfort yourself. As for our contemporaries, after a glass or two most of them are ready to spill the beans to anyone within hearing, but as the whole point of having secrets is sharing them when you shouldn't, who can blame them, especially when we'd do the same? *See also Betrayal.*

Self-employment is for those of us who are too bloody-minded to work for someone else, and who have the energy, confidence and communication skills to persuade people to use our services. As we still (I trust) have much to offer, we can either use our knowledge and expertise to become consultants, or we can become entrepreneurs *(q.v.)* and find a gap in the market to do something that nobody else is doing or, if they are, doing it better. It's risky, of course, and you have to work harder than you ever did for some company or corporation, and take all the important decisions as well as responsibility for anyone you employ. But no one can fire you, unless you do something illegal or go bankrupt, and if you've got it right, which with all your experience you bloody well should have, you'll wake up each morning looking forward to the next challenge. Or at least with a list (*q.v.*) of things that'll keep you busy.

Selfishness at our age is a way of surviving, and may also be a protection against being let down after an embittering experience. You don't get to be seriously old without looking out for yourself, unless you're a saint, and if you've reached that enviable point when you don't really care what other people think, putting yourself first comes naturally. Ideally you shouldn't cultivate selfishness to the point when no one else will come near or care for you, unless they're being paid, but it's perfectly possible to combine being selfish with judicious generosity that will encourage others to do what you want, and even love you for it.

Sex slows from a fiery tango to a stately waltz. I have never quite believed those men who say they are relieved to have reached the age when they no longer feel the sexual urge, which someone compared to being unchained from a devouring monster. Most people don't stop thinking about sex when they grow older, they just don't do it as often. That's surely not because we lack the opportunity, since most of us no longer work full time. It's because at our age consensual sex requires tact and diplomacy, and if penetrative sex is the objective, there is the real possibility of failure. Men tend to bury memories of coital catastrophe, but past disasters loom large when the equipment fails to respond to the urgent demand of its owner. Like accusatory ghosts, they can turn haunt into humiliation, which can only be banished by medical help or, better, a sense of humour. Of course, sex at our age needn't involve penetration: a good cuddle can work wonders if the partners have the time, patience and desire to please one another. And there's still time to learn something new, provided you're prepared to put aside years of reticence and actually talk about what gives each of you pleasure. Though ageing bodies slapping against each other can seem faintly ridiculous, conversation can turn embarrassment and frustration into an enjoyable experience. The most active organ in the body – apart from the heart and brain – is, after all, the tongue.

Sexism has no place in our culture or society, and those who abused their power to force themselves on people who wanted nothing to do with them sexually have lived to regret it. This isn't political correctness (*q.v.*), it's learning from experience, and though we weren't perfect, nor were most of us exploitative monsters. We who matured in the 1960s tried to behave like good guys, and if we can't modify behaviour that is now deemed inappropriate and treat people of different genders with the respect we expect ourselves, we've made no progress and should be ashamed of ourselves.

Shopping can be a treat as long as you can afford it, but people divide into those who look for something particular, and those who go shopping not knowing exactly what they want, except they know they want *something*. And there's division over the technology, of course: shopping online is so easy once you get the hang of it, I'm amazed anyone wants to spend their time and money getting to an overcrowded shop on overcrowded roads and then wasting hours dithering over what to buy, squeezing the fruit and sniffing the veg, when you can return stuff bought online if it's not to your liking. Even going into a bookshop, which naturally I support and encourage others to do, renders me brain-dead within minutes because I'm overwhelmed by choice. Of course I recognize the social value of going shopping, and though I can usually think of things I'd rather do, my curmudgeonly attitude always vanishes when I meet someone I can gossip with rather than trudging the aisles.

Sighing is something we do far too much of. We sigh when we sink into our chair and when we get out of it, when we bend over to take off our clothes and when we struggle to put them on, when we get into bed, walk round the shops, prepare a meal, or do the washing-up. It's not like puffing when you've walked up a bit of a hill, or having to take a rest because you've overexerted yourself, it's not a grunt of pain or a squeak of surprise: our sighing has become a reflex, a soft and comforting exhalation that we hardly notice. It makes us sound as if we're sorry for ourselves and bearing great burdens with noble fortitude, and we should really tell ourselves to stop it.

Singing is one of the most enjoyable ways of showing off in public, and if you're not very good at it no one will know, apart from the people on either side of you. As a leisure pursuit it is good for posture (you have to stand straight in order to let your diaphragm swell), the lungs (you have to expand them fully and breathe properly), and the brain (whether or not you can read music, you have to work out where the tune is going and how your part fits in with the others). It's sociable – a good leader or teacher attracts singers from all over the place; it gets you out of the house and helps combat stress by making you concentrate on producing a lovely noise to the exclusion of all else; when it works it's an incredibly satisfying achievement to which you all contributed; and if you're really keen, you and your group can give a little concert for an audience who may be even older than you are. And unlike a book group *(q.v.)*, you don't have to do homework unless you can't resist practising when you're alone.

Size matters, even at our age. Not your chest or your willy, but the bit in between, for starters: if it's pear-shaped you attempt to disguise it, if it contracts you worry you've got cancer. Those of us who aren't tall should have given up worrying about our height years ago, but as we all shrink as we grow older, people who haven't seen us for a while may think we're disappearing altogether. When it comes to possessions, if once we were concerned about having a bigger house/car/garden than our neighbours, now we fret over whether their largeness is too much for us to cope with. At least size is irrelevant where con-versation – the glue that holds us all together – is concerned: the tongue is one of the most active organs in our bodies and, like our hands, feet, and head, its size never alters.

Skin is amazing at restoring itself, but bruises, grazes, cuts and wounds seem to take for ever to heal at our age, even if you are accustomed to keeping yourself elastic with moisturizer (*q.v*). The unblem-ished sheen of youth becomes mottled with moles, warts, lumps, bumps, freckles and liver spots, hairs sprout in places you don't want them and cease to grow in places you do, and the veins that used to lie delicately beneath the surface now make themselves as obvious as knotted string. Lines, creases, wrinkles and furrows are all evidence of use or abuse, and while skin is marvellously accommodating when it comes to containing the parts that swell, it also sags and flakes and droops and forms folds that become tricky to clean. Of course if you can afford it you can have your blemishes sliced off, your hairs stripped, your wrinkles smoothed, and your saggy bits tightened or plumped up, but our skin is the living and inescapable testament to everything our bodies have experienced, and we should be proud of it in all its flawed but marvellous cragginess.

Sleep *see Insomnia.*

Snoring is one of the few things that inspire murderous thoughts in otherwise stable couples. Both genders snore at our age and both protest that they don't; men may snore more loudly than women, mainly when they're drunk, but they stop – temporarily, at least – when prodded or shouted at, or they wake up with a resentful 'Whatsamatter?' and, infuriatingly, fall asleep again. My wife mutters 'Sorry' when I bounce on the mattress to stop her snoring, and of course I would also apologize if I believed I was really disturbing her, though the noise is obviously made by her or the Snore Fairy. There is no effective cure other than separate bedrooms, if you

can afford them. And you can always come together
for a healing cuddle.

Solitude, as opposed to loneliness *(q.v.)*, is an
admirable demonstration of character and self-
sufficiency. I'd like to think I could manage it if I
had to, but I suspect I'd fail. Solitude means enjoying
your own company, keeping yourself entertained and
stimulated, being responsible for your own actions,
and not caring if you don't see another soul. If you've
been in a relationship and are suddenly bereaved, you
may withdraw into solitude to come to terms with your
grief, or escape the well-wishers who, however well-
intentioned, won't leave you alone. If you've never
been, or had the chance to be, solitary, it's a chance
to try something punishingly different, knowing (if
you don't leave it too long) the world will welcome
your return. If you take to it, it's fine until you have a
fall or get ill or incapacitated, and though you might
be able to rely on social services, it could be difficult
to readjust to the proximity of other human beings.
But there is something noble and antique and ascetic

about choosing solitude in a world so inextricably interconnected. You just need an inner strength not all of us possess, certainly not me.

Sport see Games.

Stinginess creeps up on us unpredictably and makes us stubbornly refuse to open our wallets or flash our credit cards, the way a horse will inexplicably refuse to jump a fence. It's not an act of prudence, like saving *(q.v.)*, it's an atypical fit of miserliness, usually provoked by outrageous prices or demands that are suddenly too much to bear. We think of it as an individual act of rebellion against crass commercialism; others will view it as mere meanness. They may shake their heads, but they will probably follow our example.

Stoicism, or fortitude in the face of misfortune, is a front we keep up for the sake of our friends and family. But while no one likes jeopardizing a reputation for strength by crumbling in a moment of weakness, there are times when we need to show that we are still capable of being scared or overcome by emotion. We need it for ourselves, because being brave all the time is too hard, and quite boring, and others need to know we're not superhuman. Or not always.

Suicide: when I was young, I thought anyone who talked about killing themselves was just seeking attention. I was wrong, several times over. Now people of our generation talk openly about suicide when they are desperately ill and have no quality of life. They don't want to be a burden to those around them, and seek an end to their suffering. The law is currently against them, but that might change. I support dignity in dying, but I learned a lesson from neighbours who told us, and their children and anyone who was interested, that they would commit suicide before they became incapable of looking after themselves. They'd been scarred by having to care for their own parents and were resolved not to hamper their children's lives. At the time, we all thought they were acting from the noblest of motives and willingly witnessed their signatures on a declaration of intent that attested they were of sound mind. We and their children were in our thirties, they were in their early sixties, and we never thought they'd do it. But they did, a few years later, and far from admiring their resolve, we and their families were stricken with grief, guilt and fury. Instead of respecting their selfless sacrifice, it was perceived as a gesture of pure selfishness. They were perfectly fit, and unlike the suicide of someone for whom life is unbearable, our neighbours' death seemed like a ridiculous waste. As it usually does, to those left behind.

Superstitions stay with even the most sceptical of us. I don't mean touching wood when talking about how healthy we feel, I mean those little hangovers from our childhood like saluting a single magpie or not walking under ladders. We invent new superstitions, too – one of mine is that if I get to a certain point on my daily walk without being passed by a car, I'll have good news from a publisher. This may have happened once, and crystallized into a superstition because I wanted it to happen again, but of course it's pure wishful thinking, as well as being an attempt to insure against disaster. It's also a belief, diluted almost to invisibility like homoeopathic medicine, in things beyond our understanding: we're a superstitious species and we keep our fingers crossed.

Surprise sustains a relationship, and can also destroy it. You can do something unexpected for your partner that makes them realize how joyful and generous you are; you can do something unexpected *to* your partner that shows you're an unreliable shit. Without surprise there's boredom *(q.v.)*, and we all know how fatal that is; with surprise come consequences, the unpredictability of which can itself be surprising. But life's a gamble, and at our age who can resist a flutter?

Survival is hard to live with if all your contemporaries have died or moved to Australia; infinitely harder if you've survived the death of a child or younger friend. You struggle to carry on, you wonder if it's worth it, even though we're all being threatened with longer, healthier lives. You grieve, and you get over your grief, because that's what survival involves, and if you survive long enough you become someone people congratulate, even venerate, not just because of your age, but because of your history. Our parents went through the losses of one or two world wars and survived, most of them with less psychological damage than seventy years of peace has inflicted on us. Survival is something to celebrate, providing it gives you more pleasure than pain. At least you don't need advice on how to survive, because you've managed perfectly well without it.

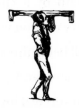

Tactlessness is something older people are good at because we don't worry much about the consequences. It's usually an impulsive expression of a view you simply can't keep to yourself – like my grandmother, who after watching me proudly change our daughter's nappy, said 'He's put it on so tight the poor child can't break wind!' – and the undeniable truth of the observation gains you admiration (though not from the wounded victim) as someone who is fearlessly outspoken. Tactlessness isn't planned, and you can always defend yourself against a charge of being outrageously rude with the line 'Did I really say that? I never meant to', as if your mouth opened all by itself.

Targets are acceptable when you set them yourself, as opposed to those pointless and useless goals imposed by ignorant interfering jobsworths. We all need something to make it worth getting up in the morning, and the trick is to aim to do something that will make a difference, if only to you, whether it's walking a little further, a little faster, or resisting the temptation to have a second helping. Some masochists like to announce their target, challenging friends and family to hold them to it, and upbraid them if they fail; those who are more self-contained keep their targets to themselves, avoiding humiliation should they falter, and enjoying private self-congratulation – which can of course be discreetly shared – when they succeed. *See also Ambition.*

Tasks see *Chores.*

Taste can set like concrete once you've passed your middle years, and only the explosive effect of a catalytic experience or new lover will make you look at things differently. We know what we like from quite early in adulthood, and our taste is formed by our desire to impress the people we respect, by our need to be different from our parents, and by what we can afford. But in maturity, where food is concerned our taste becomes limited to what's on offer, in clothes it comes down to what is comfortable, in decoration whatever we can live with is preferable to the tedium of calling in painters, and in books, pictures or records, we've collected so much we're more interested in filling gaps than acquiring anything new. Until that seismic moment when we are suddenly fed up with everything around us and want to chuck it all out and be somebody different. It may be provoked by bereavement or the need to move to a smaller place or a casual remark that makes us realize we haven't changed anything for decades. Most of us allow the moment to pass; those who don't become as contemptuous as teenagers about people who think their taste never needs refreshing. Inertia vs upheaval: I'm not taking sides.

Technology is mostly what our grandchildren handle, as they're the only ones who have the patience to enlighten us duffers. We're not Luddites: we've lived through so much technological change that has made our lives infinitely easier – the progress from coal or gas fires (or paraffin stoves) to central heating, from crystal set radios to TV on demand, from whistling kettles to microwaves, from inkwells to computers – that we are grateful rather than resentful. There are two things we *can* object to. One is the 'updates' or techno-bollocks that could only be of conceivable use to the nerds who invented it, to show off their nerdy skills and justify their nerdy salaries, which prompts the plaintive question: 'Why can't they leave things alone?' The other is the sinister abuse of technology for political ends, the manipulation of information to persuade people who think of themselves as quite savvy to believe fake facts. This heavily funded techno-propaganda employs Artificial Intelligence, bots and algorithms, and even if we're not sure what the hell that means, we have to be very much on our guard and keep warning people when they start confusing rhetoric with reality.

T

Temper at our age is like a dormant volcano: it rumbles rather than flares, but when it erupts, the lava is messy. We know from long experience that exploding in front of our loved ones is counter-productive and is either ignored or creates an atmosphere that results in indigestion and insomnia, especially when it is, as usual, our fault. And a bad-tempered outburst in front of friends merely makes us look petulant and foolish. We may be a mite more tolerant than when we were younger, and minor irritations have become part of everyday living: throwing a hissy fit won't change anything, and doesn't even make us feel much better. But just occasionally we lose it, perhaps because of an accumulation of petty irritations, perhaps out of sheer boredom or exasperation because things aren't going quite as we wanted and we're fed up with being asked what's wrong. So we blow, and because we're not used to losing control even we may tremble at the force of it. If you're lucky, your audience will feel your temper is justified; if it surprises them as much as it surprises you, you may lose a friend or be in for a night in the spare room or have the doctors check you over.

It's good to know you've still got the energy to show your temper, but it's also frightening, for you as well as them. It may be forgiven, but it won't be quickly forgotten. *See also Anger.*

Threats, as we know from bringing up our incredibly well-adjusted children, should never be uttered and then not carried out. If you threaten to withhold payment from a plumber who botched the installation of your new dishwasher until he's put it right, you've got to stand by your guns, even if he denies responsibility and threatens to call in the bailiffs, which could seriously damage your hitherto impeccable credit rating. We don't issue threats the way we used to when we were younger and cockier, and we've learned that it's usually possible to arrive at a compromise that leaves both sides reasonably satisfied. But from time to time you find yourself in a position where you're being taken advantage of, and you may have to threaten sanctions to show that just because you're old doesn't mean you're a pushover. What you have to ensure is that the threat is within your power to execute. It's no good saying you'll expose their criminal behaviour in the media if the only reporter you know retired years ago, or threatening to sue when your lawyer only handles divorces. Threats rumble in when reason has failed, and they should always be proportionate.

Tolerance is important but you don't have to go overboard. You've spent years tolerating your partner's little idiosyncrasies, like cutting their toenails in the bath, but that doesn't mean you have to welcome for dinner the first person they ever slept with, who they re-met on Facebook. You may tolerate your daughter-in-law's reactionary politics, but you don't have to stand for her being mean to your son. With grandchildren, you can tolerate pretty much anything if they're with their parents, and wait till you've got them on their own to teach them how to be responsible human beings. As for the rest of the world, I think we've earned the right to be *in*tolerant of shoddiness, knavery, lying, hypocrisy, cruelty and gross incompetence. We should, if we have the energy

and are sufficiently incensed, make clear our dissatis-
faction and offer suggestions for improvement, politely
if possible, forcefully if not. Being tolerant doesn't
mean accepting behaviour we find intolerable: speaking our mind may not make much difference, it
may (or may not) make us feel better, but we'd kick
ourselves for doing nothing.

Treats are not rewards for good behaviour: those
are bribes. Treats are little pleasures that can be
given on a whim, without any moralizing about
them being earned. No one is too old or too young
to enjoy a treat: the joy of it is in the surprise more
than the indulgence. Be generous with treats, especially to yourself.

Tremors are at best disconcerting and at worst
terrifying. You find your hand shaking when you
pour a cup of coffee, or pick up a pen to add something to the shopping list, and you're convinced
you've got Parkinson's or MS. But as the doctors will

T

tell you, tremors are a common occurrence as we grow older, often being a benign palsy that has no obvious cause – switching from ordinary to decaffeinated coffee makes little difference – and no serious effect on your general health. You may drop or spill things, and people will notice as you fill up their glasses, but unless you've ruined their clothes they should be too polite to say anything, as they will realize it's just another annoying infirmity we seniors have to live with.

Trust is something we have to rely on more and more as we get older and shakier. We've learned enough over the years to know whom *not* to trust, and if we can't rely on our family, friends and advisors to look after us and our affairs when we no longer trust ourselves to do so, it's probably too late to worry. Mind you, that trust has to be earned: my mother kept us all up to the mark and questioned – and criticized – every decision we made on her behalf until she was over 100, when she decided that as we hadn't bankrupted her or put her in a home, she might as well trust us and stop worrying. We might have wished she'd done it earlier, but it was a sweet moment nonetheless.

———

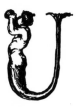

Understanding should be a cinch at our age, given the sympathy we've acquired with experience. It's sometimes hard to understand erratic behaviour in our friends – when they split unexpectedly or fly into a sudden rage – but we can ascribe that to frustration or senility. It is far harder to understand the current trend towards a culture that threatens to negate everything we value. I'm not just talking about fashion or language, I mean a political shift as profound and challenging as the one our parents lived through in the 1930s and 1940s, a mood that rejects what we call rationalism, tolerance, multiculturalism and dialogue in favour of insularity, intolerance, intemperance and hate. Is this our fault for allowing our 1960s' permissiveness to drift into indifference as politics became increasingly remote from our everyday concerns? We just wanted everyone to be themselves and make a difference, but when that didn't happen in the way we hoped, most of us shrugged and got on with our lives. The young 'new right' blame our generation as well as the baby boomers for fucking everything up, and I completely understand that feeling of fierce joy people get when someone successfully challenges our corrupt and complacent rulers. But don't the young understand the consequences of putting illiberal ideas into practice? Have they no feeling for their victims, those marginalized like themselves but of a different colour or culture? It's easy for us to sigh and say what comes around goes around, because we may not be around to see civilization growing grubby. We have to engage with those who attack our so-called liberal attitudes, and make them understand that, for all its faults, representative democracy delivers more benefits to more people than a cruel, lying, ferociously corrupt autocracy. A world without the values we've lived by

U

won't be worth living in, even if we're not here to see it.

Upbringing still seems to matter, even though our own is past mending. When a child, grandchild or friend brings someone round for your approval, you can immediately tell what kind of upbringing they've had, and though you wouldn't dream of commenting on it, unless confident they can withstand your candour, it's hard to overcome doubts if the qualities you value – manners, respect, modesty – are missing. But if you breathe a word of criticism you will immediately be accused of snobbery, and even if you try to put things right by citing examples of people with different upbringings getting on famously, you will be attacked for your old-fashioned views on class distinctions. We fight our upbringing until we are confident enough to accept it, and if you've been brought up properly you should leave it at that.

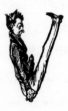

Vanity keeps us going. When we stop caring how we look, how we entertain, how we choose to impress our friends and enemies, or how we spend our money, we might as well be dead. Far from being a vice, the daily struggle to keep up appearances motivates us all. It's only when it becomes an obsession that crowds out everything else, such as a sense of proportion, that it becomes dangerous. Look at Donald Trump.

Vegetarians don't necessarily lose weight or live longer, but becoming one, especially in your maturity, is a way of surprising your friends and family,

challenging chefs to come up with something inter-
esting (the French and Russians are disappointing
as well as disappointed), and also involves the sort
of compromises that are so much a part of growing
older. I surprised my teenage daughters by turning
vegetarian after I had plucked, gutted, cooked and
eaten a pheasant shot by a friend – not because I was
squeamish, but because I could no longer condone
the killing of such a beautiful bird, after which it was
easy to give up eating anything with a face. But I still
enjoy eggs, love cheese, drink milk, and wear leather
shoes, though I tell myself they come from cows that
lived to a peaceful old age, preferably in a socialist
country. It's not a religion or a fad, it's a lifestyle that
just happens to benefit the environment, and one
that makes us feel better – not necessarily superior –
about ourselves and the world.

Vitamins are either essential to keep us healthy at
our age, or an expensive rip-off and complete waste
of time, depending on whom you believe. Despite
endorsements from wrinkled celebrities of the benefits

they derive from taking the damn things, if we've got this far surely the diet we've followed for years supplies all our needs? And as a member of that generation who were force-fed vitamins when rationing was in force – remember that sweetened orange juice, cod liver oil, and that syrupy yeasty stuff that came in a brown bottle? – I rebel against taking further vitamins on principle.

Vocabulary changes so rapidly there's little point in our trying to keep up with it. We're perfectly capable of holding a decent conversation with the words we've acquired over the years, and as with technology *(q.v.)*, if we attempt to use the new slang we're bound to get it wrong and become objects of pity bordering on contempt. Apart from political correctness *(q.v.)*, the neologisms the young use are so ugly and limited in application, they're better avoided. The language we learned is expressive, flexible, and often beautiful, and though of course it's always in a state of flux, if it's properly used it will be properly appreciated. Innit?

V

Vulnerability is not limited to those who can't take proper care of themselves. Even the strongest and most outwardly successful of us is wounded by a hurtful jibe, whether or not it was maliciously meant, and though we have developed a carapace over the years, we still bleed inside, like we did as teenagers. When in pain, what we tend to forget is that the young are even more vulnerable than we are, because they haven't had our experience and are still working out their survival strategies. So don't lash out unless you can't stop yourself, and if you do let fly, be ready with comfort.

———

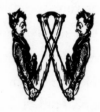

Walking is the cheapest and simplest form of exercise *(q.v.)*, assuming you're capable of putting one foot in front of the other. You don't need any special equipment or skills, you can go wherever you like at whatever speed suits your mood – the 'experts' say it should be fast enough to raise your heartbeat, yet not too fast to hold a conversation, but even ambling for half an hour is going to stretch your limbs and improve your circulation. If you're on your own you can think, if you're in company you can chat – conversation in the open is different from talking inside, perhaps because you focus on things you can see rather than abstract matters. You observe more walking than you do using any other form of transport; you can stop when you want to without worrying about parking; you can extend your distance or your speed if you want to push yourself; or you can simply stop and admire, which works especially well with a dog. You won't grow thin, but your complexion will improve as well as your fitness, and if you get bored you can always clamp on some headphones. I've seen people walking and texting or having loud conversations on their mobiles, but at our age walking offers an escape from all that, a delightful opportunity to be solitary – unless you're with the dog and bump into a fellow-owner.

Wasting time is a practice so frequently condemned by our parents when we were teenagers that now we have the leisure to indulge in it, we've forgotten how, or feel guilty even contemplating it. Which is ridiculous, as idling, or pottering about doing nothing in particular, is a valuable antidote to the puritanical drive to make every second count. We don't want to descend into sloth, which could quickly become boring *(q.v.)*, but being moderate in maturity means striking a balance between activity and relaxation, between ticking items off our to-do list and taking a couple of hours off to enjoy something that doesn't have a point. Whether that's staying in bed on a rainy day watching rubbish on TV or sloping off to the pub for no better reason than you fancy a pint, wasting time is like making compost: it's at its most productive just before it turns to sludge.

Well-being has recently become an industry. I'm aware that I'm tiptoeing into it with this Companion, which I hope will make you feel better about yourself, but I'm not promoting any products, or trying to get you to spend money (apart from the price of the book), and the only advice I offer is to be wary, which you were already. Our well-being depends on the good things we have experienced, like love and laughter, and if you've lost or forgotten those, your instinct, your friends and your common sense will surely be more effective than anyone who purports to peddle happiness.

Willpower tends to atrophy with age, when vanity loses out to laziness. But it can be defibrillated into action by a chance remark, sometimes by a child, that makes us see ourselves as others do. When our daughter was pregnant with her second infant, our young grandson patted my stomach and said, 'Baby sleeping?' I went on a diet immediately. It didn't last, but I was shocked into making the effort.

Wills should be regularly updated to take account of changing circumstances, including our own. We should also make those close to us, and our doctors, aware of what treatment we do or don't want if we develop an illness that denies us any quality of life, or if we can no longer make decisions for ourselves. It's another thing we put off, because no one likes to dwell on their own mortality, but some of the beneficiaries you named in your will may have died or forfeited your good opinion, some of the charities you wanted to help may have become mired in scandal or stopped functioning, a divorce or new relationship within the family may mean you want to reward or punish different people from those you originally envisaged. It's your last chance to show your approval in concrete terms, and provided you revise your will when you're relatively calm and relatively sane, you should get on with it.

Work/life balance matters enormously, but if you haven't worked that out by now, it's probably too late. You'll be tempted to tell other people how to organize their lives better, but unless you're a shining example of someone who got it right, they'll ignore you, as they will most advice *(q.v.)* that wasn't what they asked for.

Worrying is something we're really good at: we're anxious about our families because we know all the bad things that could happen, and we privately worry about ourselves as death and disease diminish our circle. A certain amount of stress is good for keeping the adrenaline flowing, but when it makes you feel ill or inhibits your ability to function, you have to seek help. Sharing your worries is supposed to make you put them in perspective, but your long-term partner may be so familiar with them they dismiss them or offer perfunctory reassurance, while your closest friends may listen only for a gap into which they can insert their own concerns. If you have nobody to talk to about things you feel may sound trivial but which have suddenly assumed alarming importance – your health, your finances, the fact that you haven't heard from someone you were hoping might call – you need a professional, someone who can listen impartially and offer advice objectively. You may think you've managed perfectly well without sharing your weaknesses with strangers, but worrying can be like a disease, and you need all the help you can get.

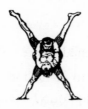

Xenophobia is irrational when a country relies on and has benefited so much from immigrants, and it makes a nonsense of the comforting idea that better education produces more tolerant citizens. But in our lifetime immigration has increased as much as inequality, and when people feel they are denied the benefits that others enjoy, the easiest thing is to blame strangers for taking what they think of as rightfully theirs. However, as nobody takes any notice of us when we point out that immigrants are doing the jobs we natives no longer want, we can only hope that if they are shut out, it will not be long before being deprived of their services will become so painful they will be welcomed back. That's optimism for you.

Xmas can be a bugger: if your children are married, they quarrel over which in-laws to invite and which to avoid; if you're alone you don't want to spend it by yourself, but nor do you want to sick yourself on a friend. If you can afford it, you could go to a hotel or on a cruise, which will be full of canoodling couples, though you might meet another solo senior. You could do something charitable like helping feed the homeless, or you could pull the covers over your head and wait until it passes. Season of goodwill and joy? Bah, humbug!

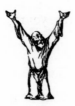

Yoga is something I admire but have never practised. I like the idea of doing exercises that relax the mind, relieve stress and keep the body trim, and those who go in for it look great and are infuriatingly calm. Of course we would all benefit from it, if we had the time. I'm going to save it for my old age.

Youth deserves our respect and sympathy. Think what we were like when we were their age, recall how little we've learned, and reflect on how much more difficult it is for them than it was for us, financially, politically and emotionally. Remember what we admired about people who are now our age – their humour, generosity, individuality, courage, their ability to listen. Even if you don't have all of those qualities, you can still be nice to the young. They might even be nice in return.

———

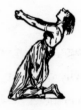

Zealots should be avoided at any age, especially if they're our contemporaries. Who needs people who lecture without listening, parade their prejudices with pride, and believe anyone who doesn't agree with them is not only wrong, but evil? It's bad enough when we come across a contemporary who has developed the missionary zeal of a convert, but it's even sadder and more dangerous when it's someone younger who might actually practise what they're preaching. Of course we must try to engage them in dialogue and get them to see reason, but with the true zealot it's a waste of breath and brain cells, unless it's your child that is involved. We can hope that there will be enough people of sense to neutralize the effects of zealotry, but that's a pious hope at best.

The *Zeitgeist*, or spirit of the age, is slippery and protean and no one knows how, why or when it will change its shape or character. Nevertheless, we have to pay it heed. We don't have to kowtow to it: of course we pride ourselves on our independent way of thinking, and ascribe our successes to being different and standing out from the crowd. We shouldn't censor ourselves, but we've surely learned the hard way that timing is as important as talent (and perseverance) in any creative endeavour, and if you're not attuned to the zeitgeist, and can't subtly adapt to its shifting codes and strictures, you risk being caught up in the crowd of its victims, and unable to persuade anyone to listen to your defence.

Zoos are a problem: a great place to take our grandchildren, but what's our moral take on keeping wild animals in cages or enclosures? There are some zoos where the animals are kept in disgraceful conditions, but of the best we can say they are places to keep rare beasts from dying out or being poached or killed, where they can breed in safety and be properly looked after with, perhaps, a view to releasing some of their progeny back into the wild. We can show our grandchildren real live animals they might only see on television, even if they travelled to their native countries, and give them the experience of touching, smelling, and learning something about them. And yet – when we took our own grandchildren to a wildlife park we came across a giant anteater, walking round and round his enclosure, obviously stressed and bored and, for all we knew, lonely and sad. We'll never know if he'd be happier in the wild, but he certainly didn't look happy imprisoned in his exercise yard. With all our experience, it's not an easy thing to explain. But then, if you've read this far, you'll know that not every question has a straightforward answer.